Simplified
Tai Chi 8 Form

A quick and easy step-by-step routine
blending Tai Chi and Yoga movements and breathing
requiring very little space and no special outfits or
equipment.

Jac Guy

No special outfits are required or recommended. Non-restrictive clothing will allow you to move easier.

Traditionally, flat soled shoes are used when performing Tai Chi but again, this is not required.

THE IMPORTANT THING IS:

Whether you're barefoot or wearing socks or shoes, make sure that you will neither slide when taking a step nor have your foot grip the ground so firmly that you'll twist your knee when attempting to move your foot.

All that you need to perform the
Simplified Tai Chi 8 Form
is a spot large enough for you to
extend your arms out from your sides,
both in front and behind you...

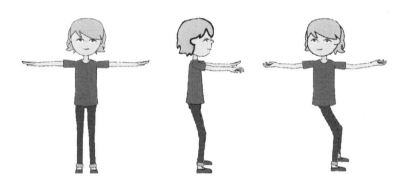

... and room to lunge to each side.

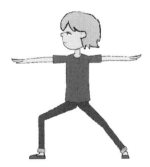

Moving From Form to Form

Moving from form to form is like an exaggerated walk.

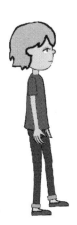

Before you step, your weight is evenly distributed on both feet.

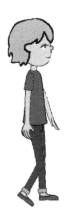

As you're about to step, you shift most of your weight to one foot as the other lifts into a Toe Stance.

For a period of time as one leg is moving, all your weight is on the other leg.

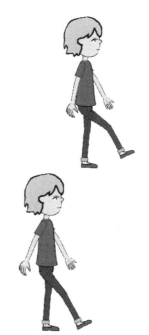

As the moving leg descends, it lands in a Heel Stance.

Your weight then shifts to the moved leg and the other goes into a Toe Stance.

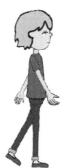

This is the simple footwork you will be using as you move from side to side.

**The side lunge is called
a Bow Stance in Tai Chi
and is a major part of the Warrior Pose in Yoga**

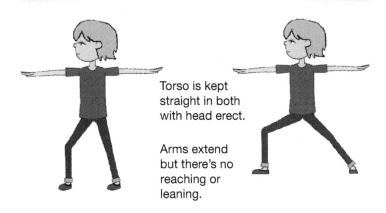

Torso is kept
straight in both
with head erect.

Arms extend
but there's no
reaching or
leaning.

In Tai Chi: feet are turned
slightly inward for better
balance. Less emphasis on leg
stretch - maintaining good
balance when stepping into
and back from the lunge is
more important.

In Yoga: feet form a T. Stance
is wider - more emphasis on
leg stretch.

When performing lunges in this 8 Form routine,
you will be concentrating on your movements
and on your breathing.
Step out only as far as you are comfortable.
Try both foot positions and use what you feel
most stable in.

*NEVER LET YOUR KNEE GO
PAST YOUR TOES WHEN
LUNGING!*

Breathing

- Inhale slowly and deeply. Exhale slowly and fully.

- Match your movements to your breathing so that you keep your movements slow and controlled.

- Keep breathing while performing the movements - don't hold your breath - unless you're underwater or in a very toxic environment!

- In general, whenever you are opening your chest - inhale. Whenever you are constricting your chest - exhale.

- When you inhale, lift your tongue to the roof of your mouth. When you exhale, let your tongue drop to the "floor of your mouth" (behind your bottom teeth). Your lips remain closed. You are inhaling and exhaling through your nose only.

Moving

- All movements are slow and relaxed as if you were just swaying in a breeze.

- Concentrate on your movements.

- Be actively aware of how it feels when you turn your head, extend and retract a limb, rotate a joint, shift your weight from leg to leg, etc.

- Your eyes will be calmly watching each hand, in turn, as it's moving, but don't focus on it so intently that you make yourself dizzy.

- Stand with feet comfortably apart and facing forward.

- Put left leg in Toe Stance.

- Lift left leg and turn to left, then lower left foot into a Heel Stance.

- Shift weight onto left leg in a shallow lunge.

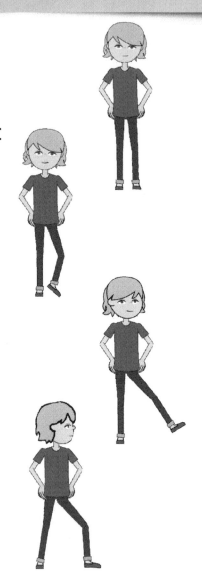

- Shift weight back onto right leg and put left foot in a Heel Stance.

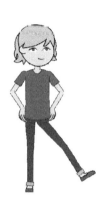

- Lift left leg and bring it back to facing forward in a Toe Stance.

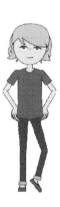

- Lower left foot and perform the same movements with the right leg.

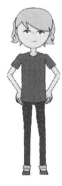

Repeat these left and right lunges until you are so comfortable with them that you don't have to think about the movement of your feet anymore than you would when you are normally walking.

Inhale slowly as you prepare to step, then exhale slowly as you lunge.

Inhale slowly as you step back from the lunge and prepare to step in the opposite direction and then always exhale on the lunge.

Before you begin...

- Clear your mind.

- Roll your shoulders back and down, elongating your neck.

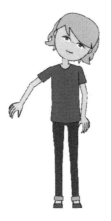 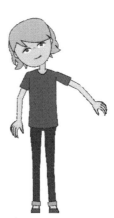

- Extend right arm and slowly & gently stretch by tilting your head to the left. Hold that position for a breath or two. Then bring your right arm in and extend your left arm and perform same to other side.

- Breathe slow and deep. Let your tongue rise to the roof of your mouth on the inhale and sink down on the exhale.

The Forms
Step by Step

Horse Stance

Commencing

Reeling Forearms

Brush Knee and Step

Part the Horse's Mane

Clouds

Rooster on One Leg

Heel Kicks

Grasp the Bird's Tail

Closing

Horse Stance

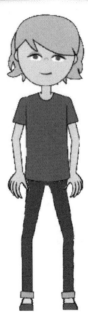

- On an exhale, left leg steps left to widen stance to about hip width.

- Torso and head stay in straight alignment.

- Shoulders are down. Arms relaxed at sides.

- Knees slightly bent.

- You should feel as if you could maintain this pose for hours and wouldn't lose balance if bumped.

- Take as long as you need to get comfortable in this position, breathing slow and deep and concentrating on how your body feels.

Commencing

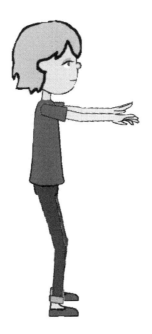

- Inhale as you slowly raise your arms straight out in front of you to about shoulder-height.

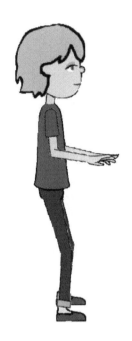

- Exhale as you let your arms drift down to about waist-height, leading with your elbows.

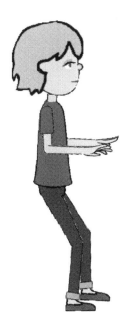

- In preparation for your next move, bend your knees a little bit more so you can comfortably turn your torso further.

Right Reeling Forearm

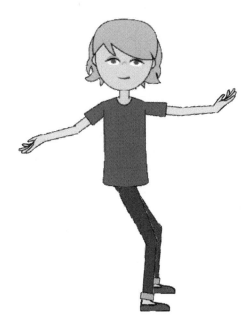

- Turn your torso to the right and your palms up.

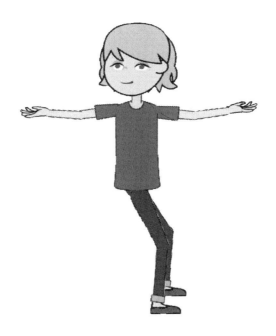

- Inhale as you stretch your arms out and raise them to shoulder-height. Turn your head towards your right hand.

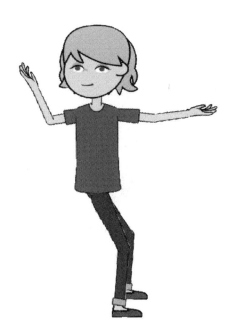

- Begin to exhale and watch your right hand as you bend your right elbow.

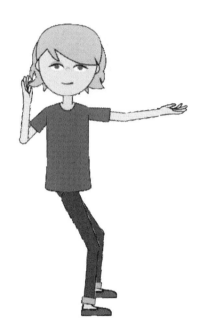

- Bring your right hand past your head.

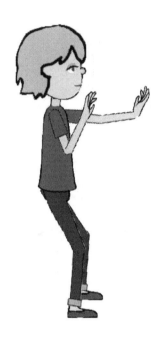

- Your torso returns to front and your left wrist curves so that your left palm is facing you.

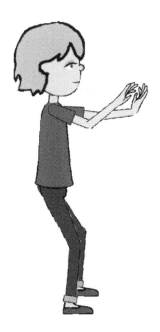

- Your right palm is brought close to your left palm but doesn't touch.

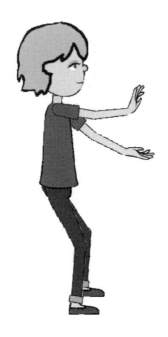

- Right palm rises and left palm drops downward.

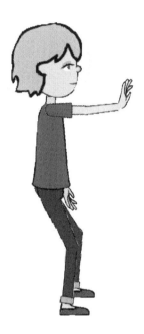

- Left arm drifts down to your side and right arm Is extended forward, palm out as if you're directing traffic.

Left Reeling Forearm

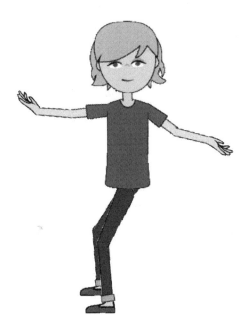

- Turn your torso to the left as your left arm circles down before turning both palms up.

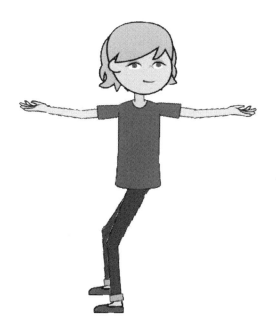

- Inhale as you stretch your arms out and raise them to shoulder-height. Turn your head towards your left hand.

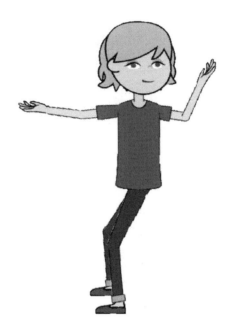

- Begin to exhale and watch your left hand as you bend your left elbow.

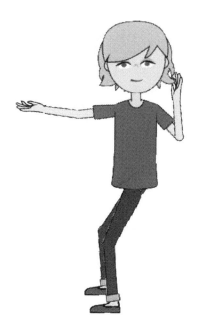

- Bring your left hand past your head.

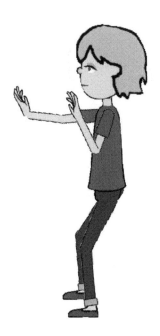

- Your torso returns to front and your right wrist curves so that your right palm is facing you.

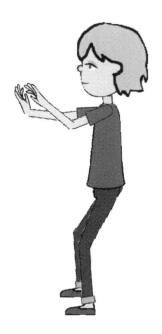

- Your left palm is brought close to your right palm but doesn't touch.

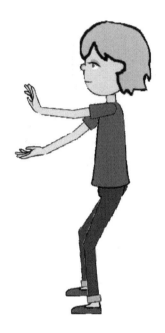

● Left palm rises and right palm drops downward to about waist-height.

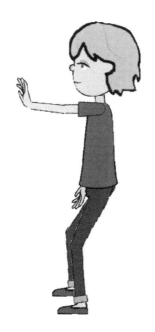

- Right arm drifts down to your side and left arm is extended forward, palm out as if you're directing traffic.

Brush Knee and Step Left

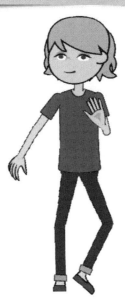

- Shift your weight to your right leg and bring your left leg into Toe Stance.

- Right arm circles down and out towards right side.

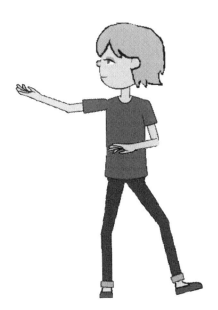

- Left arm drifts down until forearm is across waist with palm down.

- Inhale as you extend right arm out, palm up, to shoulder-height.

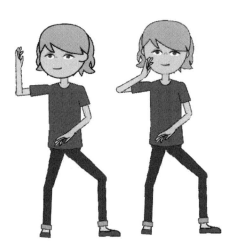

- Watch your right hand as you bend right elbow and bring your right hand past your head.

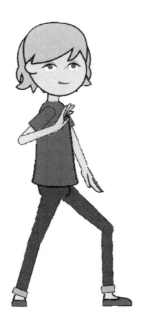

- Exhale as you turn your torso left and lunge left with left leg.

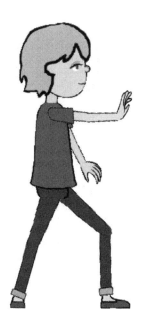

- Left hand pushes down from waist, across left thigh and out from left side, palm away from body.

- Straighten right elbow and extend right arm with wrist bent back, palm away from you.

Brush Knee and Step Right

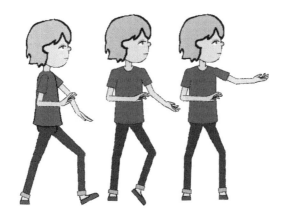

- Shift your weight back onto right leg and bring left leg in from lunge as you return your torso to front.

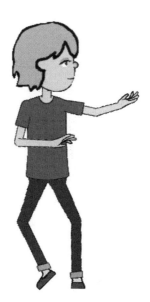

- Shift your weight to your left leg and bring your right leg into Toe Stance.

- Inhale as your right arm drifts back so that forearm is across waist, palm down.

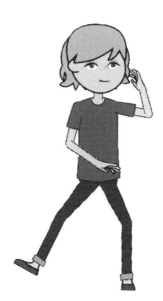

- Watch your left hand as you bring your left arm up to shoulder-height, then bend left elbow and bring your left hand past your head.

- Exhale as you turn your torso right and lunge right with right leg.

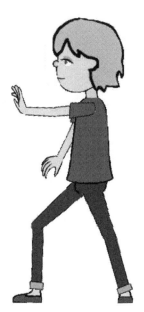

- Right hand pushes down from waist, across right thigh and out from right side, palm away from body.

- Straighten left elbow and extend left arm with wrist bent back, palm away from you.

Part the Horse's Mane - Left

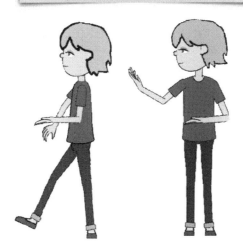

- Left arm retreats to across waist, palm up as you bring in right leg and return torso to front.

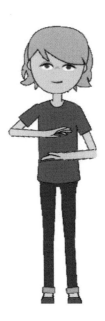

- Inhale and watch your right hand as you curl your right arm in a circle until it hovers above your left as if holding a ball.

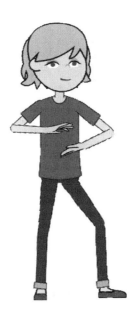

- Exhale as you lunge left with left leg and slide left hand out from under right.

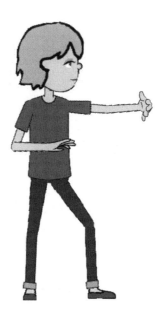

- Extend left arm with wrist curved so that your left palm is facing you.

- Right arm lowers to waist, palm down.

Part the Horse's Mane - Right

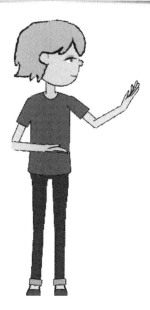

- Right arm stays at across waist but palm turns up as you bring in left leg and return torso to front.

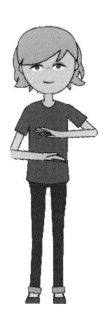

- Inhale and watch your left hand as you curl your left arm in a circle until it hovers above your right as if holding a ball.

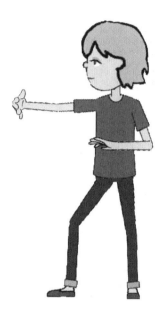

- Exhale as you lunge right with right leg and slide right hand out from under left, extending right arm with wrist curved so that your right palm is facing you. Left arm lowers to waist, palm down.

Clouds - First of Six - Left

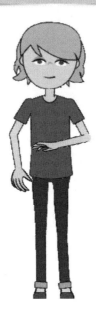

- Inhale and let right arm drift down until right palm is facing right hip as you bring in right leg and return torso to front.

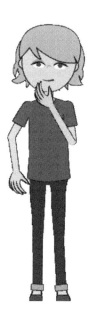

- Left palm turns toward your torso and rises to in front of your face.

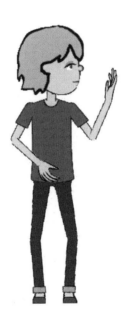

- Bend knees a bit more as you will be turning just your torso.

- Exhale and watch your left hand as it leads your torso to the left, as far as is comfortable.

Clouds - Second of Six - Right

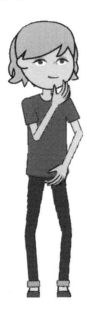

- Bring your right palm up your torso until it is in front of your face.

- Let your left hand drift down until palm is facing left hip.

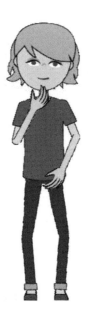

- Inhale and watch your right hand as it leads your torso back to the front.

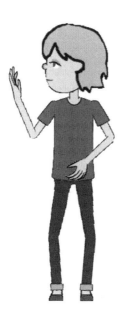

- Exhale as you continue turning your torso to the right as far as is comfortable.

Clouds - Third of Six - Left

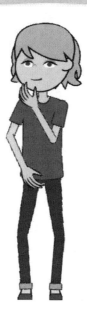

- Bring your left palm up your torso until it is in front of your face.

- Let your right hand drift down until palm is facing right hip.

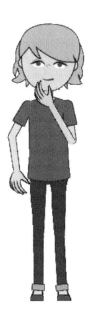

- Inhale and watch your left hand as it leads your torso back to the front.

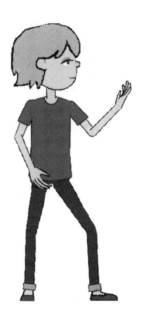

- Exhale as you continue turning your torso to the left. This time you will also lunge left with left leg. Keep following left hand to the left as far as is comfortable.

Clouds - Fourth of Six - Right

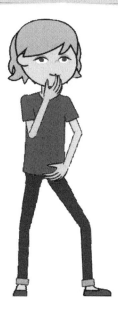

- Bring your right palm up your torso until it is in front of your face.

- Let your left hand drift down until palm is facing left hip.

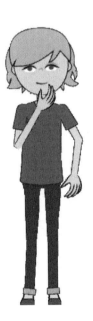

- Inhale and watch your right hand as it leads your torso back to the front and return your left leg to front.

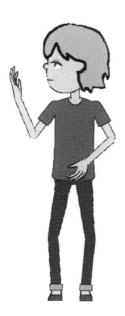

- Exhale as you continue turning your torso to the right as far as is comfortable.

Clouds - Fifth of Six - Left

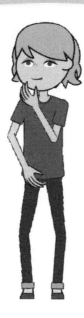

- Bring your left palm up your torso until it is in front of your face.

- Let your right hand drift down until palm is facing right hip.

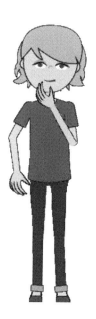

- Inhale and watch your left hand as it leads your torso back to the front.

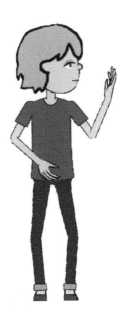

- Exhale as you continue turning your torso to the left as far as is comfortable.

Clouds - Sixth of Six - Right

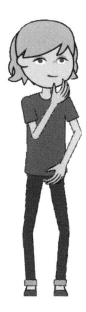

- Bring your right palm up your torso until it is in front of your face.

- Let your left hand drift down until palm is facing left hip.

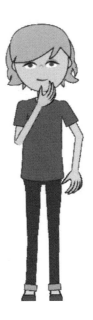

- Inhale and watch your right hand as it leads your torso back to the front.

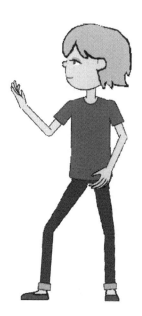

- Exhale as you continue turning your torso to the right. Lunge right with right leg. Keep following right hand to the right as far as is comfortable.

Segue from Clouds to Rooster on One Leg

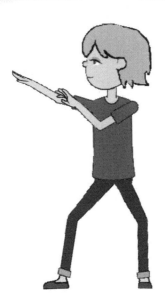

- To segue into next form: inhale and let both arms drift upwards to your right, palms down. Left palm rises to about shoulder-height and right palm is a little higher.

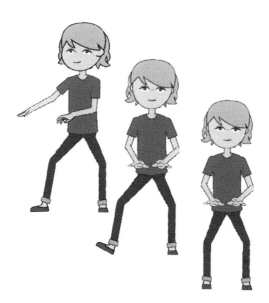

- Bend your knees for a brief shallow squat as your hands swoop down and to front on the exhale, ending with palms down at waist-height as you rise, bring in right leg and turn torso to front in Horse Stance.

Rooster on One Leg - Right

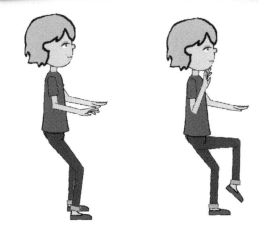

- *You can either pause at this point with your right leg in Toe Stance before beginning the Rooster Form or you can move right from the segue swoop into standing on your left leg.*

- Inhale and bend right elbow so that right palm is facing away from you at about shoulder-height.

- As you raise your hand, also raise your right leg. Let your right foot dangle toe down. (Try to bring your knee up to your right elbow - but not touching - without leaning forward or losing your balance. If that isn't possible yet, just try to keep your foot off the ground.)

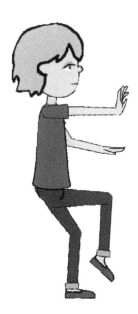

- Exhale as you straighten your right elbow
  out in front of you.

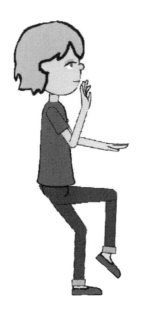

- Then bend your right elbow, allowing your hand to retreat back towards your shoulder.

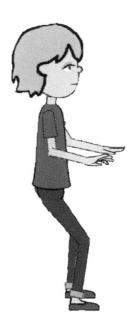

- Lower your right palm down to waist-height and your right leg to floor simultaneously.

Rooster on One Leg - Left

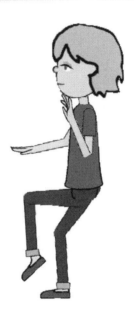

- Inhale and bend left elbow so that left palm is facing away from you at about shoulder-height.

- As you raise your hand, also raise your left leg. Let your left foot dangle toe down. (Try to bring your knee up to your left elbow - but not touching - without leaning forward or losing your balance. If that isn't possible yet, just try to keep your foot off the ground.)

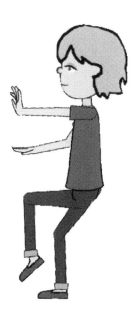

- Exhale as you straighten your left elbow out in front of you.

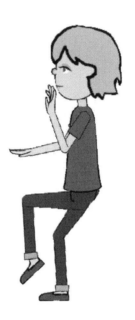

- Then bend your left elbow, allowing your hand to retreat back towards your shoulder.

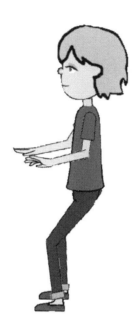

- Lower your left palm down to waist-height and your left leg to floor simultaneously.

Heel Kick - Right

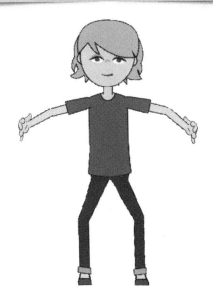

- Inhale as you raise both arms up and out from shoulders.

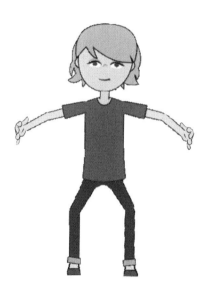

- Exhale as you bend your knees and drop into a short squat - keep torso straight - don't lean down.

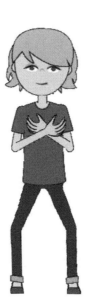

- Bring arms down and towards your torso so that your palms are facing you and your wrists are crossed - left wrist closer to you - right wrist on outside.

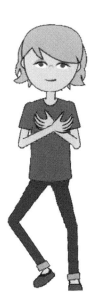

- Inhale as you stand and shift your weight to your left leg - right leg goes into Toe Stance.

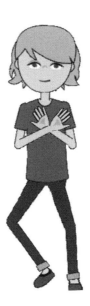

- Turn your palms out, facing away from you.

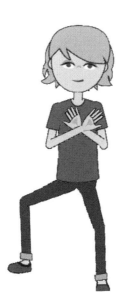

- Flex your right foot up and raise your right leg.

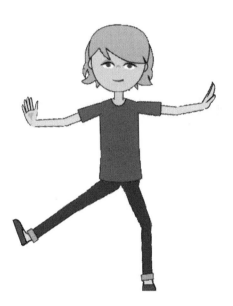

- Exhale as you straighten your right knee so that your leg is diagonally extended from your right hip. Don't snap kick. Keep your movements slow and controlled. Try to extend the leg from hip height but if that isn't comfortable yet, just try to keep your right foot flexed and off the ground.

- As you extend your right leg, also extend your arms out. Your left arm can be straight out from your side but your right arm extends diagonally forward parallel to your right leg.

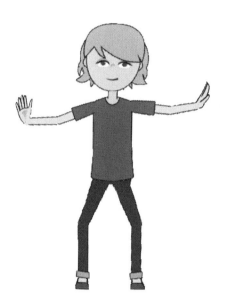

- Inhale, leave arms extended but bend right knee and return right foot to the ground.

Heel Kick - Left

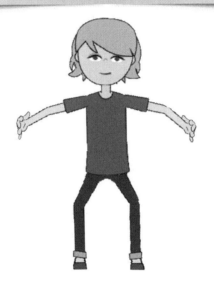

- Turn hands so palms face each other and exhale as you bend your knees and drop into a short squat - keep torso straight - don't lean down.

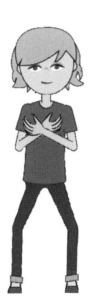

- Bring arms down and towards your torso so that your palms are facing you and your wrists are crossed - right wrist closer to you - left wrist on outside.

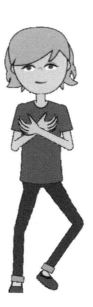

- Inhale as you stand and shift your weight to your right leg - left leg goes into Toe Stance.

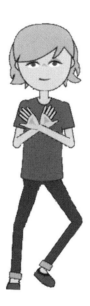

- Turn your palms out, facing away from you.

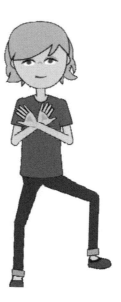

- Flex your left foot up and raise your left leg.

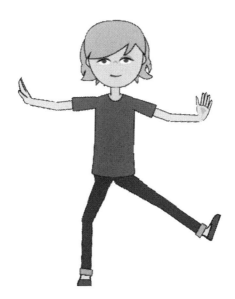

- Exhale as you straighten your left knee so that your leg is
  diagonally extended from your left hip. Don't snap kick. Keep
  your movements slow and controlled. Try to extend the leg from
  hip height but if that isn't comfortable yet, just try to keep your
  loft foot flexed and off the ground.

- As you extend your left leg, also extend your arms out. Your
  right arm can be straight out from your side but your left arm
  extends diagonally forward parallel to your left leg.

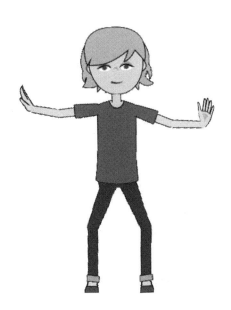

- Inhale, leave arms extended but bend left knee and return left foot to the ground.

Grasp the Bird's Tail - Right
Part 1 of 4

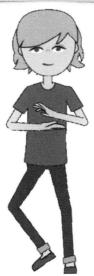

- Inhale as you bring right arm down in a curve so that your forearm is across your waist, palm up.

- Curve left arm so that it hovers above right arm with palm down. (Make the ball.)

- Right leg moves into Toe Stance.

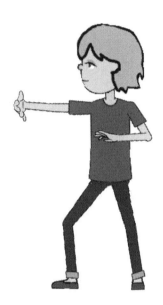

- Exhale as you lunge to right and extend right arm with wrist curved so that your right palm is facing you. Left arm drops to across waist, palm down. *(Identical to the Part the Horse's Mane form).*

Grasp the Bird's Tail - Right
Part 2 of 4

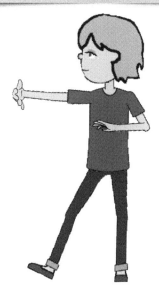

- Inhale as you shift your weight back on your left leg and put your right leg into Heel Stance.

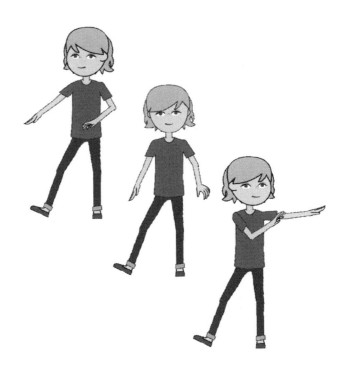

- Both arms drop down and gently swing up in an arc - the left extended out from left shoulder - the right forearm across chest, hand at left shoulder, palm down.

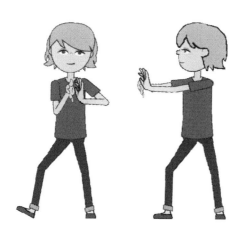

- Exhale as you bring your left hand with fingers pointed upwards to your right palm which is held sideways. Push against your right palm as you shift your weight back into a lunge to your right.

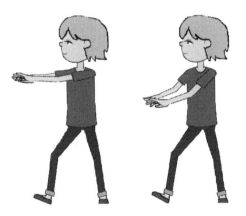

- Turn both palms down and inhale as you shift your weight back onto your left leg, putting right leg in Heel Stance.

- Arms retreat back towards torso at waist-height.

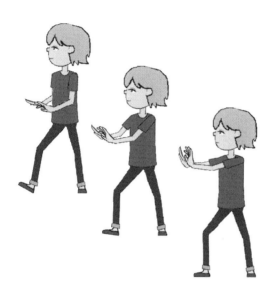

- Exhale as you push both hands slightly down then out from chest as you once again shift weight onto right leg in a lunge.

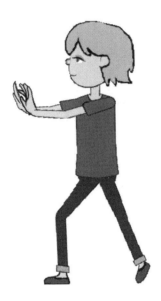

- This time you end the move by bringing your left leg up into a Toe Stance.

Grasp the Bird's Tail - Right
Part 4 of 4

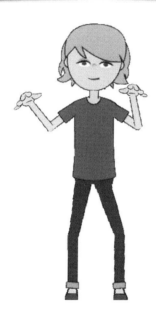

- Inhale as you turn torso back to front and bring right leg in.

- Arms remain extended out from chest, palms down and swing with torso as if floating over a huge globe.

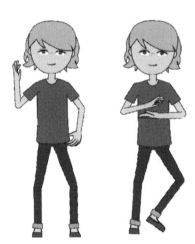

- Maintain the circular movement as left arm drifts down to waist-height and turn palm up.

- Right arm bends at elbow to hover over left with palm down. (Make the ball). Left leg moves into Toe Stance.

Grasp the Bird's Tail - Left
Part 1 of 4

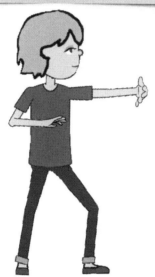

- Exhale as you lunge to left and extend left arm with wrist curved so that your left palm is facing you. Right arm drops to across waist, palm down. *(Identical to the Part the Horse's Mane form).*

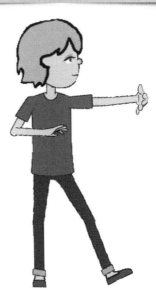

- Inhale as you shift your weight back on your right leg and put your left leg into Heel Stance.

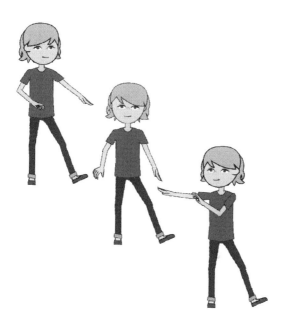

- Both arms drop down and gently swing up in an arc - the right extended out from right shoulder - the left forearm across chest, hand at right shoulder, palm down.

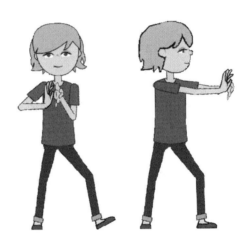

- Exhale as you bring your right hand with fingers pointed upwards to your left palm which is held sideways. Push against your left palm as you shift your weight back into a lunge to your left.

Grasp the Bird's Tail - Left
Part 3 of 4

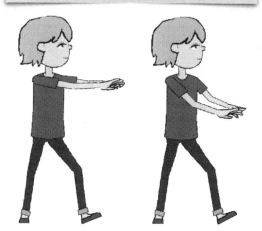

- Turn both palms down and inhale as you shift your weight back onto your right leg, putting left leg in Heel Stance.

- Arms retreat back towards torso at waist-height.

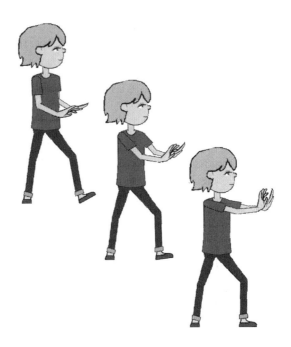

- Exhale as you push both hands slightly down then out from chest as you once again shift weight onto left leg in a lunge.

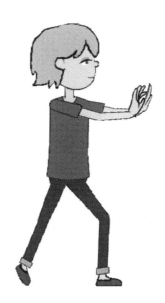

- This time you end the move by bringing your right leg up into a Toe Stance.

Grasp the Bird's Tail - Left
Part 4 of 4

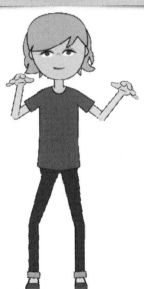

- Inhale as you turn torso back to front.

- Bring left leg in and turn left foot so it faces front.

- Arms remain extended out from chest, palms down and swing with torso as if floating over a huge globe.

Closing

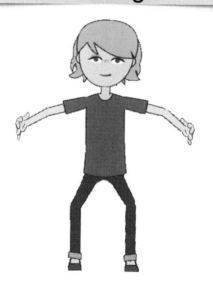

- Exhale as you bend your knees and drop into a short squat - keep torso straight - don't lean down.

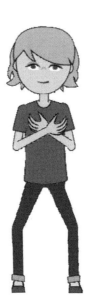

- Bring arms down and towards your torso so that your palms are facing you and your wrists are crossed - left wrist closer to you - right wrist on outside.

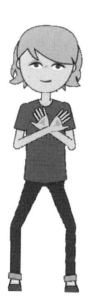

- Inhale as you stand and turn wrists so palms are facing away from you.

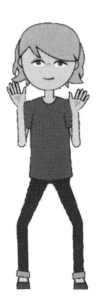

- Move hands out to shoulders.

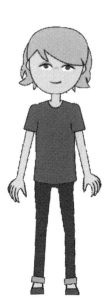

- Exhale as you lower your arms to your sides and bring left leg in.

Final Thoughts

Here are 2 tips you may wish to try to make learning this routine easier:

1. Perform one form correctly every day for a week and then each following week add on another form. For example: in week #1 step into Horse Stance and perform the Commencing moves. In week #2 step into Horse Stance and perform both the Commencing and the Reeling Forearm moves. In week #3 add the Brush Knee and Step…you get the idea.

2. Remember: no one will come knocking on your door to punish you if you practice these forms in mirror image! You will be performing each exact move to both the left and the right so it really doesn't matter which direction you start with.

Thank you for trying this Simplified Tai Chi 8 Form. I hope you enjoyed it and that it brings you comfort.

If so, you might also enjoy a "Stand in Place" symmetrical Tai Chi 24 Form which is currently in the works.

Here's to staying happy and healthy!

Printed in Great Britain
by Amazon

36451427R00073